DR FRAY ANDREA

HOW
WEIGHT LOSS
WORKS

REVEALED SECRETS ABOUT WEIGHT LOSS

Table of Contents

INTRODUCTION

This book is meant for changing your body to the physique you want. In doing so, you will end up being the better version of yourself, one who is fit for accomplishing any objectives in your day to day existence. Could it be said that you are attempting to shed pounds while managing diabetes? "On the off chance that you have excess weight, losing even 5% of your body weight can emphatically help your wellbeing. Weight loss can further develop your glucose levels as well as can bring down hypertension, coronary illness chance and, surprisingly, how much medicine you take," says **Dr. FRAY ANDREA**

I began my own personal growth journey by first changing my body from a condition of "weak and soft" to a strong and lean physique. While doing this, I understood the force of this change. In addition to the fact that I was seeing an improvement in my body. I was more ready, sure, and hungry to get what I truly needed throughout everyday life.

I before long understood that by accomplishing this extreme objective for myself, which requires all that I have, I turned into a totally different individual, a better version of myself inside and out. Presently I can unhesitatingly say that I am more disciplined, more tireless, and more clarity of mind. I started accepting that this is the sort of person I'm presently.

Individuals generally act in a way they accept addresses what their identity is. In the event that you are an individual of high discipline, you will act in a like manner. At the point when your psyche advises you to remain at home and not go to the gym, one more voice inside you will say, "I'm going on the grounds that I am focused and this is the proper thing to do."

At the point when you practice this discipline again and again, whether it be going to the gym, hitting the treadmill, or eating the right things, **YOU** become a trained individual since you have imbued this habit into your tissue, your being. This is the sort of person you are currently. From here onward you can apply this conviction and conduct to some other parts of your life and further develop it. How would you think this will influence you in accomplishing your objectives?

I accept you ran over this book which is as it should be. It may be the case that you are looking for something, something to advance your life, regardless of whether you know it intentionally. The way that you are perusing this presently is a sign — a sign you should go on with. Pay attention to your internal receipt, your premonitions, and not the negative contemplations that you are barraged with more often than not.

Toward the finish of this book I want to believe that you will find a portion of the responses you were searching for.

En route I want to believe that you understand that this book is about far beyond changing your body. It's truly about figuring out who you truly are also. Just keep in mind, your everyday habits will decide the existence you need or don't need. So pick shrewdly to make a propensity that will get you what you need and not the alternate way.

Chapter 1: REASONS Before RESULTS

1.1 *You Should Have a Strong For what reason to Accomplish Your Objectives*

What is a strong WHY? How might I have strong Why's? For what reason do we want to be strong? Why's? Have you at any point had an objective you didn't accomplish? I sure have. Have you at any point asked why you didn't accomplish it? Have you at any point accomplished an objective and wondered why you accomplished it?

Addressing these inquiries will permit us to find those strong WHYS we want to succeed. So what are your strong Why's?

Those strong For what reasons are different for each individual. Your strong For what reason may not be a strong WHY for someone else. For instance, one strong WHY for me was to excel at discipline by going through the body change process. I realize you need to teach yourself a great deal of things you might like to do all through this excursion. That's what I understood on the off chance that I can teach myself to find true success in this field, I can find actual success in others too. This might be a strong WHY for me, yet not really for someone else. Being focused may not mean quite as much to them as getting the physical make-up they need. To get to your strong Why's, you should not waste time in writing down every one of the motivations behind why you believe you should do this. For what reason would you say you will do specific things to get it? When you have around 10 or 20 reasons, select your top five, the "MUST" haves for you to do this.

1.2 - What Are Your Genuine Reasons? Inward Objectives versus External Objectives

Is your objective for weight reduction just to look great to dazzle others? Or on the other hand is it for you to see yourself in the mirror and say, "I love the manner in which I look and I feel great"?Both are to change your body, yet both have altogether different inspiration levels. I can perceive as a matter of fact that the last option is a greatly improved driver than the first.

Keep in mind, assuming we do it for ourselves, the fire is a lot greater than if we endeavor to do it for another person.

Have you at any point recommended to somebody that they ought to stop smoking? How has everything turned out? Not even specialists can advise a patient to stop smoking. By the day's end, it will depend on that individual and no other person to choose to at last stop for their own reasons.

My point here is that you should do it for your own reasons. Do it since you need to improve personally, to arrive at your maximum capacity, to be fit so you can do any open air exercises you need effortlessly, to be enthusiastic so you can play with your children the entire day. Those are the reasons that won't be the ever finishing fire that consumes each hindrance en route. These are your inward game reasons.

External game reasons like looking great, squeezing into a hot garment, or dazzling somebody are great, however they will not have that enduring power. Trust me, in the event that your only object is to change your body for these external game reasons, it will be a battle and you may not come as far as possible.

Allow me to pose you a conspicuous inquiry. How simple is it to change your body? Not extremely simple is it? In actuality, it could be quite possibly the hardest thing you can do in the course of your life. It requires extraordinary inspiration, tolerance, and ingenuity. I feel that is the reason when you accomplish this marvelous objective, all the other things become more straightforward.

I would not joke about this. You will ask yourself, "Wow on the off chance that I can do this, what else I can do?" In the event that you were effective in arriving at one objective before, you will probably arrive at numerous different objectives since you have the experience and teaching to make it happen. Furthermore, you can rehash it and again as long as you need.

1.3 How to Remain Spurred With Your "MUST" WHY's

When you have your rundown of "MUST" reasons, you are prepared to go after your objectives. This is your wood to the fire to move you along. It's anything but a question of if, yet when.

At the point when those difficult stretches come and you want to stop, take out this rundown and read it again and again until it sinks in and you feel certain.

The "MUST" reasons typically influence you

also, your friends and family. So having this promptly accessible will give you the lift you truly need. Ask yourself, is it adequate to let yourself down as well as your friends and family too? I realize this might appear as though you're by and large too unforgiving with yourself; in a way you are, yet remember, we are here to come by results. It's anything but a stroll in the park.

There will be hindrances, obstacles, and openings we need to get around.

I accept the explanation we ask ourselves these

"WHY" question is on the grounds that we're keen on whether it is truly helpful for us. We ask ourselves, "How might this benefit me" all the time since it's incorporated into our DNA for endurance purposes.

So we ask ourselves, "For what reason would it be advisable for me to eat things I abhor without a doubt?" or "For what reason would it be a good idea for me to run on the treadmill when I could be staring at the

television?" or "For what reason would it be a good idea for me to go to the rec center when I can stay in bed?"
The main individual who can answer these
questions are you. The main individual who can Take care of business." Therefore we want an extremely strong and convincing motivation to get things done, particularly in the event that things are unfamiliar to us or awkward.
So once more, ask yourself..."Why would it be advisable for me to get in shape?" Record every one of the advantages in the event that you shed 10 pounds, 20 pounds, 30 pounds, or more. How might you respond? How might you feel? Envision it.
Could you feel more certain? Could you have more energy? Would you love life more? Could you have a more energized outlook on the day? Could you feel that you could be wrong? Could you offer more consideration and love to your loved ones?
Getting thinner is tied in with making yourself more joyful inside for you, not for any other person.
The sooner you understand this, the sooner you will get your butt moving. It's about you. It's tied in with cherishing yourself and offering yourself the consideration we as a whole need and merit. At the point when you know about this and acknowledge liability regarding yourself and the manner in which you feel, accept me, things will begin to change in a fantastic manner.
Here is an imbecile inquiry. How could you
Do you need to encourage yourself? Have you at any point posed yourself this inquiry?

It's senseless I know, yet attempt it. It will as a matter of fact give you greater clearness regarding your end objective.

Model: I need to feel more joyful inside so I can communicate it outwardly. At the point when I'm cheerful and alive outwardly, I will cause others around me to feel the same way.

That is clearness! Presently the inquiry is, do you want that? I surely do!

What's the other option? Could you rather feel hopeless, pushed, simply attempting to endure the day? Obviously NOT.

In the event that you're perusing this book, you certainly try not to need that. You are the sort of individual who needs sure change in your life, and you ought to be glad for that.

Congratulate yourself and say, "I am pleased with myself. I'm gaining ground toward making the existence I need, and I realize I can get it done". Truly, I believe you should quit pursuing and truly say it, without holding back if conceivable.

Presently, how would you feel? Truly, don't you feel a marvelous good energy flooding through your body? Do you feel that certainty? On the off chance that not, say it over and over until you really do feel it.

Listen to this; not at all like a great many people, I would rather not simply endure the day. I need to experience the day to its fullest, appreciate it, and encourage others simply by being around me. I realize you need this as well, and that is the reason you're perusing this book. Or then again perhaps you simply needed to lose some weight. One way or another, I couldn't care less; you've coincidentally found this book and it is my obligation to assist you with improving your life than at any other time, the most effective way I know how — through wellness!

At the point when you begin to get more fit, you will have an incredible outlook on yourself. Your mind gets going and takes care of you with lots of good considerations that will support your certainty.

At the point when you have more certainty, you will believe you should do more things that will make you feel much better about yourself. This is what wellness truly gives you. Indeed, the side-effect is a hot, hot body, yet more so your outlook moves forward another level. You will start to ponder everything since you put stock in yourself as well as other people. It's fundamentally similar to you've been given another pair of glasses forever, and when you glance through the focal points, you perceive how incredible things truly are.

1.4 Deal with Yourself First, then, at that point, Others

The main thing is the reason you make it happen. I do it since I find that being in the rec center or simply practicing gives the energy, the inspiration, the certainty, and the psychological durability I want to handle different pieces of my life. If I have any desire to be in charge of my life, the outcomes I get are conscious, not unintentionally. Preparing yourself every day of the week, you become a restrained individual. That's what presently takes and applies the discipline to different aspects of your life and see what occurs.

Assuming you've gotten this far, I know you don't as a rule mess around with rolling out an improvement in your life, and that begins with your actual wellness.

Assuming you've at any point gone via plane, you've likely known about the airline steward going over the wellbeing strategies not long before the plane takes off. Do you review when he declares that when the air veil drops from a higher place, ensure you put it on yourself first before you put it on your kids? This appears to be legit, right?

You're not decent to anybody assuming that you're dead, correct? I realize this is a solid piece, however this is reality. You should deal with yourself, your body, your brain, and your soul first.

Then you reserve the option to deal with others. Don't briefly imagine that you're being narrow minded when you contemplate dealing with yourself first and attempting to work on yourself to improve personally.

From my own insight, I can tell you that when you attempt to work on yourself and become better, certain individuals, including your own relatives, won't comprehend and will express things to stop you.

"For what reason do you want to get thinner?" "Who are you attempting to dazzle?" "This isn't significant; bringing in cash is." Don't pay attention to that poop, regardless of whether it's from your own loved ones. Eliminate yourself from circumstances like this and listen

just to your inward voice. Hear just that voice directing you in the correct course for you.
You understand what you're doing. You have a rundown of motivations behind why you're changing yourself...it's so you can better yourself and give more to other people. Like inspiration, positive energy, and backing. Kindly let me know how this is narrow minded. I say this since I've been called out previously. Anticipate it and acknowledge it, however don't give it any power.
Pass on it with the mists and keep on seeking after the body you need so you can have a superior life.
To end this chapter, we should turn out some of the things on which to make a move:

1.Write down on a piece of paper as many reasons as you can for why you need to lose weight . For you also, for other people. Compose no less than 10 reasons.

2.Keep it with you and read it ordinarily before you start your day. Peruse it around evening time as well, if possible.

3.Share your objectives with your cherished ones and request their help.

Do this currently prior to continuing on toward the following part. Pick one thing and do it consistently, then intend to do the others the next day.

Chapter 2: Mindset

2.1 Positive Mental Demeanor versus Negative Mental Demeanor

So what does mindset have to do with losing weight? For my purposes, this is everything.

Your mindset will decide your result. Meaning in the event that you want to make it happen, you will. The equivalent is additionally evident in the event that you figure you can't. Henry Portage once said, "Whether you want to or you can't, you are correct."

In chapter one you concocted every one of the motivations behind why you want to change your body. You thought of them down so you can involve them as gas for your inspiration. It will give you that push you want to get through any sort of obstructions and self restricting considerations. Did you have any idea that as people, we normally return to pessimistic reasoning more often than not on the off chance that we don't make ourselves suppose emphatically? I've unquestionably

seen this all through my change. Tragically, we are recently wired that way, yet luckily we can take care of that. We can just supplant our negative contemplations with positive ones and continue to zero in on them. At the point when that's what you do, the negative contemplations will vanish on the grounds that our brains can hold just a single idea at a time.

Positive mental disposition is significant in light of the fact that we want this main impetus to get us to the furthest limit of our objective. Negative considerations will cloud us and shut down our excursion on the off chance that we don't supplant them with positive contemplations. At the point when we are in a negative outlook, we lose our drive and inspiration to continue onward. Contemplations like 'It's excessively hard,'

'For what reason am I burning through my time?' and 'This is truly not so significant,' will begin to populate your brain. You should kill these contemplations by focusing on certain considerations for a while. Center around what you need, the ultimate objective. You want to propel yourself by continuing to persuade and empower words consistently .

Peruse your attestations. It's trying to drive your psyche to think positive thoughts constantly, however in the event that you can continue to make it happen, soon you will develop another propensity for thinking. What's more, that propensity will remain with you forever.

2.2 Norms and Convictions

Presently we really want to request one of the main inquiries in this journey.

Could I at any point do this? What's your response? I trust it is, "Heck, definitely I can!"

First you Should accept that you can make it happen. You should have an immovable conviction that you can make it happen. On the off chance that you accept you can make it happen, you will track down a way, and things in the universe will adjust to assist you with arriving. You really should accept you can make it happen and be persuaded that you will get to the furthest limit of your objective since, in such a case that you don't have confidence in yourself, who will? Unquestionably not your neighbor or any other individual.

Here is a decent tip to use to assist with your conviction. Ask yourself, do you know anybody or have you known about any individual who has shed 10 pounds, 20 pounds, 30 pounds? Isn't that right?

The response to this question is obvious! There are loads of individuals today who have had the option to lose 10, 20, 50 pounds or more. This is a reality. In the event that they can make it happen, for what reason mightn't? They're worse than you are, they're not more astute than you are. Then, at that point, what is halting you? The main thing that can stop you is yourself. Your negative considerations and restricting convictions will annihilate your fantasies and objectives.

Absolutely never let this occur. Harbor just certain considerations that you can make it happen and you will track down a way, regardless. At the point when you harp on steady considerations like this, your brain will not have space for the negative ones to come in. This takes a great deal of training, however you can make it happen. Once more, what's the other option? An unfulfilled life, an existence of disappointment that you didn't take the plunge, an existence of not as much as what you merit. Is this OK with you? I would like to think not.

Certifications: To assist with boring the positive convictions into your head and body, record five announcement articulations to help you. Take a gander at them each day and night to move you along.
Here are a few models:

1.I can do anything I set my attention to.
2.If they can make it happen, so can I.
3.I have limitless potential.
4.I am focused on accomplishing my objectives regardless of anything.
5.I decline to pause and nothing can stop me.
6.I will get up each time I fall.
7.I won't ever surrender.
8.Failure isn't a choice.
9.I won't ever fizzle since I will try constantly.
10.I have every one of the assets I want to succeed.

2.3 - Start In view of the End

Ask yourself what it is you truly care about. Be extremely clear and record what you need; the way to arrive will begin to unfurl for you. You won't see things you on earth might have seen previously — everything that will assist you with arriving at your ultimate objective.

That is the way amazing our brains are. In part one, we recorded why we needed to shed pounds. Presently we want to know what precisely it is that we need, the subtleties.

1.What is your optimal weight?

2.What is the wellness level you need?

3.Do you need an athletic form, lean areas of strength for and?

4.Do you need a long distance runner's fabricate? Slim, deft, inconceivable perseverance.

5.Do you need a weight lifter's physical make-up? Solid and solid.

You should be totally clear on what sort of body you need on the grounds that the way to arrive is marginally unique for each objective.
How would you conclude which body type you need?
Permit me to share my experience. For my purposes, It was tied in with bettering myself so I can do what I truly appreciate doing. I appreciate being in the exercise center and lifting loads. I appreciate sorting out like a jock. I appreciate gaining ground in how much weight I can lift. On the other hand, I additionally appreciate exercises like climbing, playing tennis, participating in any sort of sports, and running.

So for me it was tied in with consolidating weight training with the outside. I need a physical make-up that can lift loads yet additionally be extremely utilitarian in doing exercises about which I'm enthusiastic. The body type I held back was nothing like the Wellness Model Look. This body type is decently strong, however not so large that you're cumbersome and can't squeeze into standard apparel. You're exceptionally practical and coordinated. You're sufficiently able to lift a few decent loads and can float through the outside exercises without a perspiration. You great search in a suit however under your life systems diagram.

I find this body type works for me. So presently that you know how I made it happen, put in almost no time recording what body type you need. Once more, be as unambiguous as possible.

This will help your objective proceed. One thing I believe you should make note of is that this objective isn't established. By this I mean your objectives might change as you progress in this way, and that is absolutely alright.

My underlying objective was to get fit so I could do different things effortlessly. I never figured in 1,000,000 years that I would need to contend in weight training. Objectives change since we become somebody unique, somebody better than the individual we were the point at which we began. Simply recollect, you are allowed to alter your perspective, your objectives.

Caution: Simply don't do it since it is easier...never do this.

I would not joke about this. A simple way is a way not worth taking.

Alright, presently we understand what we need exhaustively. We have an unmistakable concentration. How would we arrive? In the following section I will impart to you every one of the essentials of shedding pounds and the systems to assist you with arriving. All I want from you is the obligation to make a move. Bargain?

Chapter 3: Losing Weight

In the past chapter we discussed mindset and how we really want to trust that we can succeed, be extremely clear on what we need, and start considering the end. To get to your definitive objective, you should make moves constantly. Little ones and large ones, it doesn't make any difference. What makes a difference is practicing the movement on a regular basis to draw you nearer to your objective. What I found functioned admirably for me was to have little wins consistently, regardless of whether it was something minute, such as recording my goal for the afternoon. These little wins could be perusing my assertions each day...it truly doesn't make any difference. The point here is to construct a propensity for doing something without failing to arrive at your objective. At the point when you recognize these little wins, you will be certain that you can make a move each and every day. Before long you will make increasingly big moves until you quickly track your direction as far as possible. This is known as a Propensity Compounding phenomenon.

How would we make these little wins consistently? What moves do we make?

3.1 - Picking apart

To figure out what basic assignments I ought to do consistently, I figure out my objectives.

This is just a method delineating every one of the fundamental stages to get to your objectives. First you would record your objective, then record every one of the exercises, then focus on them by arrangement and significance, then, at that point, continue to separate the exercises until you get to the easiest errand conceivable.

Whenever you have delineated every one of the significant stages, recognize the most straightforward assignments and make time in your schedule to do one to three things day to day. This way you will understand what to do and not need to consider it.

It's truly about making it simple for you to make steady everyday moves. On the off chance that you know what to do, when to do it, and how to make it happen, it's an issue of utilizing your self discipline to act. That is all there is to it. Assuming that the activity is not difficult to do, it doesn't take a lot of resolve to make it happen.

Doing this consistently will ultimately practice it regularly, very much like awakening and cleaning your teeth, and it will presently not be something troublesome to do. Keep in mind, things are troublesome before they become simple. Expect this and continue to do it until it gets simple to do.

Presently you have lucidity on what you really want to do each and every day. The reality of understanding what to do will give you the certainty you really want to accomplish your objectives. Lucidity is power. At the point when we don't have this, we feel befuddled, baffled, and demotivated on the grounds that we aren't sure about our bearings.

The main thing I do in the first part of the day is get exceptionally clear on my objectives and the basic errands I want to do that day. Then I shut out an opportunity to make it happen. I sort out my errands by grouping and need. Grouping includes figuring out which errands should happen first before the others. By need includes what has the most effect on your objectives. Then I approach doing them, never continuing on until one is finished.

Tackle the main errand first and concentrate until done. In the event that you don't follow through with the responsibilities on that day, move them to the following day and go on until the undertaking is finished. By doing this, I generally finish the main errands first prior to continuing on toward the less significant assignments.

Attempt this strategy for using time productively and efficiency; remain at it and see what works out. I guarantee you it's completely phenomenal. You will amaze yourself whenever you've arrived at your objective and ask yourself how you did that.

3.2 - Little Day to day Habits

One critical component to being self-inspired is to make little day to day propensities and do them consistently. At the point when you do this, you are accomplishing something consistently — winning.

The greater part of us likes to win and accomplish; I realize I do. At the point when this occurs, we become more headed to continue onward until we arrive at the ultimate objective. How does this apply to getting in shape? For me it was just about as basic as drinking four liters of water consistently and going to the exercise center each day, whether for lifting or cardio. I did this for such a long time that when I didn't go to the rec center for only one day, I could feel the impact, similar to something that was absent.

Have you at any point gone every day without your wireless? Gone every day without drinking espresso? Or on the other hand something different that you do consistently? It's exactly the same thing. It's WITHDRAWAL from your everyday propensities since you've incorporated this action into your daily practice and presently it's a piece of you. On the off chance that you do without it, in any event, for a day, you will feel the unfriendly impact right away. My point here is that it's exactly the same thing with practicing and eating right to get thinner. When you become familiar with practicing consistently and following what you eat, it will end up being a propensity and you won't have any desire to let it go.

Take me, for instance. I actually track my macros on MyFitnessPal on my telephone pretty much consistently on the grounds that I did it such a huge amount during my prep for rivalry that it is presently my propensity and part of me. At the point when I eat something it's generally in my sub-conscience to figure out the amount I'm eating or what sort of food I'm placing in my body.

Presently I'm not saying that you will get this way and turn into all fanatical about what you eat, however basically you will consider it.

Over the long haul you will quite often settle on choices that help your objectives.
Presently you might share with yourself, "Practicing consistently is definitely not something simple. That is hard.
How might I squeeze practicing into my life each day?" Consider the possibility that I let you know that you really want to practice for just 10 minutes consistently; how about you do that. Obviously you can. Individuals dream or sit on the latrine for 10 minutes consistently. Presently, that is a senseless correlation, indeed, yet I needed to make a point that little wins needn't bother with being a hard thing to do. Matter of reality, it ought to be something simple, essentially for the initial not many weeks and until you have made the propensity. The possibility of little wins regularly is to make a propensity. Whenever you've made a propensity and you do it consistently, such as cleaning your teeth (I truly trust you clean your teeth consistently), the propensity becomes what your identity is and afterward it is not difficult to do. Assuming that it's not difficult to do, you will be less hesitant to make it happen. Do you follow me? By doing the simple errand consistently, you will get to your objective. That is the recipe; sort out the simple thing to do consistently and do it until you arrive at your objective. That is all there is to it!

3.2 .1 Calories In versus Calories Out

The critical central to weight reduction is the rule of calories in versus calories out. The basic thought is that how much food you eat versus how much energy you consume will decide if you get more fit, remain a similar weight, or put on weight. For our weight reduction objective, we want to eat less calories than we consume. So how would you eat less calories than you consume?

First you need to decide your upkeep caloric prerequisite, otherwise called your All out Day to day Energy Use(TDEE). This is the number of calories or how much food you want to eat to remain at the same weight.

Note that it isn't urgent to be definite; you simply need a ballpark number so you can

have some place to begin. then, at that point, make changes as you come. Since you have your support number, you want to eat not exactly that add up to get in shape. What number of less calories would it be advisable for us to eat? To decide this, increase your support number by 15%. For instance, assuming my upkeep number is 2000 calories,multiplying by 15% would give me 300 calories. Take 2000 and deduct 300 and you will get your shortfall caloric admission number of 1700 calories. Eating 1700 calories will make a shortfall where you're eating less calories than your upkeep; consequently, you will get more fit over the long run.

There are multiple ways of eating less calories than you consume. The one I use is the large scale supplement following strategy. I use MyFitnessPal and track the amount I eat consistently by recording the macros, carbs, protein, and fats. An application is additionally accessible on iPhone and Android gadgets. I know some of you probably shouldn't do this and find counting calories an excess of work. That is alright; we can utilize another strategy. My other most loved strategy is dividing. Envision an ordinary size supper plate. All your food ought to fit on that plate; that is all you're eating for that feast. A big part of your plate ought to be vegetables, one quarter ought to be protein, and the last quarter ought to be carbs. This will rise to 100 percent of the food on your plate.

For instance, I like to eat Costco's sweet kale salad for veggies, so 50% of my plate is covered by salad. For protein I like to eat simmered chicken bosom, so I segment it to cover one fourth of my plate. The last quarter is covered by a yam.

This model shows you a low-fat, moderate-protein and carb diet. For the assert age individual, this is a reasonable feast to consume fat and get in shape. In the event that you're a jock or a trying contender, I would exhort that you track macros since you want a more exact number.

3.3 - Fantasies and Trends

There are numerous fantasies and trends connected with getting more fit and consuming fat. There are innumerable eating regimens and exercise projects to

allure you to purchase. These projects are made to target individuals who are searching for a
convenient solution, something simple to manage without an excess of work.
I concede that I have made it happen. It's in our tendency to find the fastest and least demanding way imaginable. This is in our developmental mind and that is fine. Be that as it may, when you know about this and can change this manner of thinking, you should do as such for your own advancement, to arrive at your maximum capacity. Try not to let this perspective break you.
What are the legends and prevailing fashions in the wellbeing and wellness industry?

•Try not to eat sugars

•You can lessen fat in a particular spot.

•You want to take enhancements to get in shape.

•Eat high protein and high fat.

•Eat-anything you-desire diet program.

There are so many more out there. The point here is to recognize that this is reality. There are loads of organizations promoting these kinds of items to individuals. You need to avoid them and never get involved with Simple. Nothing replaces difficult work, commitment, and determination. All that about getting in shape is learnable and doesn't need to cost you dearly. There are numerous assets that talk reality; you simply must be more persistent in exploring and tracking down them. Books and book recordings are an incredible beginning.

*3.4 - Good judgment versus Normal Practic*e

We truly needn't bother with a unique eating routine or exercise program to change our bodies. We really understand what we ought to do; now and then we simply need a little assistance getting everything rolling. Fortunately there are lots of assets out there, very much like this digital book, to help you on your way.
We as a whole realize that we ought to eat less broiled food varieties like french fries, and sweet food varieties like frozen yogurt, cake, and confections, yet we do it in any case. That is entirely fine; the key thing is to track down an equilibrium. I suggest an 80/20 rule for eating. The vast majority of the time eat great, healthy food and the other 20% of the time, you can eat anything that you want. This works for myself and I figure it will work for you in the event that you allow it an opportunity and stick with it for 30 days.
The method involved with changing our bodies can be simple in the event that we do it for quite a while and it turns into our way of life. Other than that, there is a difficult road ahead. All things considered, it's a test you

can defeat with a tad bit of innovativeness, discipline, and penance.

You have it in you; trust me, we as a whole do. We simply have to quit rationalizing and make a move day to day! We know what to do, and on the off chance that we don't, we can learn. Simply choose, set a due date, and make a move.

Moronic inquiry for you. On the off chance that you put $5 in the bank and toward the year's end your profit from venture was $100, could you be blissful? Obviously; I would. Give $5 and get $100 back. That is an incredible profit from the venture, wouldn't you say?

Presently what's more significant? Cash or your body?I expect you said your body.

In the event that you didn't, this isn't an ideal book for you. Your body is your sanctuary. Without great wellbeing and state of being, you can't appreciate anything cash can purchase. So doesn't it appear to be legit to deal with your body like it's your best speculation of all time?

Rather than cash, put in the right food and activities consistently to develop your body. Consequently, your body will compensate you ten times for your venture by becoming more grounded, better, and more adaptable, permitting you to appreciate all that life brings to the table and to help other people. You have sound judgment; presently utilize normal practices like practicing and eating right to get where you need to be.

Chapter 4: Mechanics of Losing Weight

This chapter will provide you with an essential comprehension of food, preparing, and cardio. I have included numerous supportive connections for more data.

The main part of changing your body is that you should have opposition prepared.

It tends to be anything from utilizing your own body weight, to lifting loads, to utilizing groups and such. By the day's end, I need to work out my muscles. In this way, any kind of preparation that makes your muscles work harder than they regularly do by applying strain and stress is fine. It doesn't need to get muddled; pick a basic strength preparing program you like and go with it. You can continuously change the program in the event that you need something different later on.

To assemble more muscle, you must go to the gym and lift a few significant burdens. Simply make sure to begin slowly, and progress gradually to stay away from wounds.

To utilize all the more a novice's preparing program, I would prescribe P90x. All you need to do is follow the program's activity and nourishment rules. Pick a preparation program you appreciate and anticipate doing consistently. As far as I might be concerned,

That was P90x. Man, I cherished it. The teacher, Tony Horton, is wonderful, so spurring and funny. I would anticipate returning home after work so I could prepare consistently. I accepted that the outcomes would come as long as I adhered to this
program strictly. Adequately sure, they did. Unprecedented outcomes, may I add. I lost
more than 20 pounds north of a 90-day time of preparing and eating right. You also can get
These sorts of results assume you find something you like and stick with it. The great part is that subsequent to doing this for 90 days, the routine turns into a piece of you
furthermore, you go on with it. You won't feel totally astounded and ever need to return to your old self.
It's similar to having an opportunity to eat at a
exquisite café that has three Michelin stars and faultless help, then returning to an eatery that has no stars and fair help. Which would you like?
I know, it's another senseless inquiry, yet genuinely apply this similarity to your body. It's
like you at level 10, with lots of energy and
cherishing life contrasted with you at level 3 with low energy and battles to endure the
day. Which adaptation of "YOU" do you like? Obviously, you are at level 10. This is my
long approach to letting you know that when you change yourself and become truly
What's more, intellectually fit, you would never need to return to your previous self. I sure didn't. I love who I'm

presently contrasted with me 10 quite a while back. You, as well, will feel this.

As you progress through your preparation and eating right, you'll see the outcomes and love it. This gives you the certainty to keep going, and afterward you will see more outcomes also, acquire certainty. Before sufficiently long you will go up to this point, you will not perceive the individual who began this excursion. This habit turns into a way of life for you — looking extraordinary, feeling perfect, and doing incredible things.

This is where I need to see you go. I maintain that this should be your way of life since you will love the upgraded you and you will go for greater What's more, better things. You won't make due with less.

You have just a single body, one lifetime, and one individual who can deal with it...YOU.

You understand common decency. Decide to do the right thing and not the simple thing. You will appreciate substantially more achievement assuming you decide to experience along these lines.

4.2 *Sustenance*

In quest for the body you need, I'd have to say that sustenance is above all else. Assuming sustenance is lord, practicing is sovereign. In the event that you ace sustenance, you are ensured the physical make-up you need.

What do I mean by dominating sustenance?

Is it hard? Might I at any point make it happen?
Dominating sustenance in this sense implies monitoring what you eat and why you eat the things you eat.

For this situation, we are eating to get more fit. We need to comprehend what we eat and

Why do we eat it? For instance, how could we need to eat earthy colored rice over white rice? A speedy Google search uncovers that brown rice is better for you. For weight reduction purposes, it assists keep you full for a more drawn out timeframe, so you don't have to eat as much. It's additionally brimming with nutrients and supplements when contrasted with white rice, which has been deprived of its supplements through the handling stage.

You can find a wide range of sustenance books and digital books to assist you with grasping food, particularly the food that assists you with losing weight and being great.

Nourishment definition: The most common way of eating the right sort of food so you can develop appropriately and be solid.

At the point when we separate food, we have large scale and miniature supplements. Full scale supplements are the sugars, proteins, and fats, while miniature supplements are nutrients and the cell reinforcement properties of food. I will not go over a lot exhaustively, however enough so you can get to your objectives. There are straightforward carbs and complex carbs.

White pasta and entire wheat or entire grain pasta would be models. Fundamentally, any carb that is white in variety is normally a straightforward carb, meaning it gets processed rapidly, giving you quick energy however not supporting totality for a really long time. A complex carb will take more time to process, however will keep you full longer.

Knowing the distinctions between them, this is the way I use them for some good weight reduction results. I eat straightforward carbs later in a strength instructional course so I can have fast energy to recuperate from exhausting movement. Your body is exhausted after extreme preparation, so you'll have to take care of what needs quick, subsequently straightforward carbs. As a model, I eat rice cakes, any natural product, or Rice Krispies bars. I pick low-fat, straightforward carb food. I consolidate straightforward carbs with protein just after my exercise to amplify muscle amalgamation — muscle maintenance.

Protein is basic. Simply eat white meat more often than not. Why? Generally white meat sources are lower in fat. Actually we don't need to eat a lot of fat on the grounds that most food varieties have fat in them. We really want almost no fat in our eating regimen contrasted with carbs and protein.

My decisions are chicken bosom, white fish like tilapia, and ground turkey. I every so often will have extra-lean meat and ground meat also.

Most specialists suggest eating in any event

your body weight in grams of protein for ideal muscle maintenance and fat misfortune. So in the event that I weigh 150 pounds, I will attempt to eat around 150 grams of protein. Protein is the building block for our bodies and muscles, so we want to protect them while we lose fat. The more muscle we have, the more calories we can consume, which will lead to the deficiency of more weight.

Fats. I observe that it is exceptionally simple to eat how much fats we want in our customary food varieties today. This is the least of my concerns. I don't actually need to make a good attempt to eat how much fats I require every day since all that we eat has some fat as of now. For instance, when we cook, we utilize olive oil; that is fat. Entire eggs have a lot of fats. Anything, truth be told, unless you purchase 0% sans fat food. Simply eat lean proteins and you'll hit your fats requirement.

4.3 - Cardio

Cardiovascular preparation is a vital part of the general intention to get more fit. Not only does this sort of preparation consume the most calories in a single exercise, it likewise demonstrates your heart and perseverance level. Having a steady cardio routine alongside your obstruction preparing and diet is essential to augmenting fat misfortune. Cardio essentially assists you with consuming more calories,

and that implies a more profound shortfall, which equivalents weight reduction.
There are an assortment of cardio practices you can look over, and each will help you arrive at your objectives another way. For purposes, the cardio we need to zero in on is consistent cardio and focused energy span preparation (HIIT).
Consistent cardio is strolling or running at a slow speed, around 65% to 70% of your maximum exertion. HIIT preparation consists of two parts. One is full-out, most extreme, 90% to 100 percent exertion for a brief period, similar to 15 to 20 seconds. The subsequent part is a sluggish, 10% to 20% of most extreme exertion for 30 to 60 seconds.
HIIT preparing consumes a ton of calories inside a short measure of time. What's more, it reinforces your heart and lungs and can assist with your weight training.
For consistent cardio you can utilize a treadmill, step walker, bike, or curved. The decision is yours. I wind up blending between the circular machine and the track factory and a sluggish run outside when the weather conditions license. For HIIT preparing, I utilized running and the curved machine.
Stir it up. Do the exercises you appreciate and that can bring results. You can have both. This way you'll keep on making it happen and accomplish incredible outcomes.
The motivation behind consistent cardio is to consume calories, for the most part from fats and carbs, instead of your well deserved fit muscle. We try not to believe that should happen in light of the fact that muscle keeps our

digestion high so we can consume more calories. Absent a lot of lean mass, we would consume not many calories as We move around or work out. That is the reason protecting muscle is so significant when shedding pounds. Also, we need to strength train and eat sufficient protein to guarantee that we keep all the muscle we can.
From my experience, doing any sort of consistent cardio a few times each week What's more, one HIIT preparation for seven days will do wonders for weight reduction. Alongside proper eating and strength preparing, this will assist with accelerating your fat misfortune.

4.4 - Enhancements

The last piece of the chapter is flexible. We aren't guaranteed to require it. In any case, it helps us. The legitimate nutrients and supplements can assist us with recuperating better, and that implies better exercises, which implies improved results. There are a couple of supplements I would suggest. Get yourself a fair multivitamin, omega fish oils, and vitamin D. I accept these are the least to assist you with your exercises.
As a contender, I take these everyday to help
work on my presentation and capability.
•multivitamin
•omega fish oil
•L-ascorbic acid
•vitamin D

•glucosamine (for joints)
•glutamine

CONCLUSION

I want to congratulate you for making it this far before we come to an end of this amazing voyage together. This demonstrates your commitment to learning and striving for excellence. Given the numerous distractions you encounter every day, your ability to finish this book demonstrates your discipline. Because of this, I am confident that you are devoted to changing.

As soon as you finished this book, I urged you to take the first step toward getting the body you wanted by writing your goals down on a piece of paper. This is an essential action that will give you the drive and assurance to keep working toward your goal every day.

So, how do you feel at this moment? Are you eager to build the body you desire, followed by the life you desire? I really do!

Statistics show that there are two sorts of individuals in terms of how they act after reading a book. One type will put the book down after finishing it and take no further action. They won't do anything. I don't know why some people act in this way, but we must learn to live with it. The other type of person will do something; they will apply what they've learned and take action.

The question is, what type of person are you? I hope you are the type who will stop talking and take action.

You are ready! Go out there, do your best, and forget the rest. Go for it and never stop until you reach your goal and nothing can stop you! The only thing you will lose is your old self and body fats!.

CONCLUSION

www.ingramcontent.com/pod-product-compliance
Lightning Source LLC
LaVergne TN
LVHW020606160826
845677LV00020B/3990

* 9 7 9 8 8 4 8 0 4 5 3 3 8 *